Charlotte Woods

the complete
Blood Sugar Diet
cookbook

easy delicious recipes for fast
weight loss and great health

**Calorie
Counted
Low Carb
Recipes**

Contents

Breakfast Recipes

Lunch Recipes

Dinner Recipes

Desserts

Introduction

Are you ready to lose weight and improve your health with healthy eating?

Sugar plays havoc with our weight and our blood sugar balance, which results in many health issues, but is it really enough to cut out sugar from your diet? Sugar is harmful but in this book we take it a step further and reduce carbohydrates to help you lose weight and restore balance to your body. Sugar and carbohydrate consumption doesn't just cause obesity and pre-diabetes, it has been linked to a myriad of illnesses. However, there is one simple and important step you can take and that is to balance your blood sugar which will help you to lose weight and achieve better health!

This book contains clear, concise information on how to balance your blood sugar by using the principles of low carbohydrate, sugar-free eating which is proven to help you re-balance your body. In this book we bring you plenty of delicious, innovative, calorie-counted recipes to make life simple and easy while you lose weight and improve your health while eating foods you thought would be off the menu. A winning combination for your health and your taste buds. It really can be that simple!

Getting In Control of Your Blood Sugar

Every time we eat our blood sugar rises and later falls as the short term effect of our food wears off, creating a cycle of peaks and troughs throughout the day, causing hunger and the desire to sustain energy levels. The ideal way to achieve balance is to avoid highs and lows by avoiding foods which cause a fast fix of energy i.e. sugar in all its forms and starchy carbohydrates. Often we are unaware of symptoms until a sudden medical diagnosis. The effects of excess sugar and high insulin levels range from mild to severe and the emotional to the physical. It has been linked to:

- Irritability, anxiety, mood swings, poor concentration, insomnia and depression.

- Fatigue, particularly after eating.

- Palpitations, shakiness and light headedness.

- Increased signs of ageing.

- Obesity, pre-diabetes and type 2 diabetes.

- Hypertension, high cholesterol, heart disease and strokes.

Virtually anyone can benefit from a sugar-free diet but be sure to check with your doctor before embarking on any radical changes to your diet, particularly if you have an existing medical condition.

Getting Started

Avoiding sugar and refined carbohydrates is beneficial, especially if your diet includes concentrated fruit juices and ready-made meals containing hidden sugars, but is your diet already healthy and you're finding you still can't shift that extra weight? Setting your personal goal is a fundamental step, so decide what you want to achieve – is it to lose a few pounds or are you aiming for increased vitality and better health?

You can either remove sugar and starchy carbohydrates from your diet or if you want to maximise the benefits you can additionally restrict your calorie intake. If you choose to limit your calorie intake, aim to consume no more than 1000 calories a day. Reducing your calorie intake will improve weight loss and if you have excess belly fat it is a great way of getting rid of this more rapidly which will have an even greater beneficial effect on your blood sugar.

Once you've decided how you want to approach your new health regime you can get started straight away. Familiarise yourself with what you can eat and remove temptation foods from your cupboards.

What You Can Eat

REDUCE or AVOID the following:

CARBOHYDRATES

- Bread
- Cereals
- Cakes
- Muesli
- Cookies
- Crackers
- Rice cakes
- Oat cakes
- Pasta
- Noodles
- Rice
- Millet
- Potatoes
- Sweet potatoes

FATS

- Vegetables oils such as corn and canola.
- Spreads and margarines which are low fat, contain trans fats or contain sugar.

SUGARS

- Avoid products containing sugar, syrup, honey, chocolate, sweets and candy. Marinades and ready-made sauces sweet chilli sauces, ketchup, barbecue sauce, and any dressing containing sugar. Always read the labels as sugar is frequently added where you least expect it.

- Avoid dried fruit, like apricots, sultanas, raisins and figs.

DRINKS

- Steer clear of beer, wine, spirits, cordials, fruit juices, sugary drinks.

Below is a list of food you can enjoy.

PROTEINS

- All meat; beef, chicken, lamb, turkey, pork.

- Eggs

- Fresh fish such as tuna, haddock, cod, anchovies, salmon, trout, sardines, herring and sole. Shellfish such as prawns, mussels and crab.

- Tofu

- Nuts and nut butters

- Seeds

- Beans and pulses such as kidney beans, butter beans, chickpeas (garbanzo beans), pinto beans, cannellini beans, soy beans and lentils.

FATS

- Butter

- Avocados

- Coconut oil

- Olive Oil

- Ghee

- Nut butter

- Full-fat dairy produce; cheeses, Greek yogurt, sour cream, clotted cream, mascarpone, crème fraiche, fresh cream.

FRUIT – MAXIMUM 2 PIECES OF LOW SUGAR FRUIT PER DAY

- Bananas
- Blackberries
- Blueberries
- Apples
- Apricots (fresh)
- Cherries
- Grapefruit
- Plums
- Kiwi
- Kumquat
- Lemons
- Limes
- Melon
- Oranges
- Peaches
- Pears
- Pomegranate
- Redcurrants
- Strawberries

VEGETABLES

- Root veg; such as parsnips, beetroots and carrots in moderation, as they have a higher carbohydrate content.
- Leeks
- Broccoli

- Cabbage

- Lettuce

- Celery

- Asparagus

- Artichokes

- Aubergine (eggplant)

- Bean sprouts

- Peppers (bell peppers)

- Broad beans

- Cabbage

- Runner beans

- Mushrooms

- Spinach

- Spring onions (scallions)

- Cucumber

- Courgette (zucchini)

- Radish

- Kale

- Cauliflower

- Pak Choi (Bok choy)

- Onions

- Brussels sprouts

- Rocket (arugula)

- Olives

- Watercress

DRINKS

- Tea

- Coffee

- Green tea

- Water

- Almond Milk

- Soya Milk

- Double cream (heavy cream), coconut oil or butter can all be added to drinks.

DRESSINGS & CONDIMENTS

- Fresh herbs and spices such as; bay leaf, coriander (cilantro), chives, mint, thyme, rosemary, basil, parsley, oregano, cinnamon, cumin, mustard, dill, garlic, ginger, turmeric, paprika, cayenne pepper, chilli powder/ flakes, pepper and sea salt.

Top Tips

One of the biggest challenges you will face is avoiding the added sugars and carbohydrates in processed foods, even those which are advertised as healthy can be loaded with sugar or be carb laden which will unbalance your blood sugar. Below is a list of suggested alternatives to make meal times and food preparation easier.

- Substitute rice for cauliflower rice which can be adapted to suit your main course by adding herbs, spices or vegetables.

- Pasta is notoriously high in carbohydrates but a portion of courgette 'spaghetti' is a wonderful way of providing a filling and delicious alternative and it can be served alongside meat dishes and casseroles.

- Mashed potatoes are a traditional favourite but a low carbohydrate mashed cauliflower with a dollop of fresh butter, salt and pepper is a great alternative which kids love.

- Fizzy drinks can be replaced by fruit infused water which is simple to make by adding a small quantity of chopped fruit to a jug of water, adding flavour plus vitamins to regular water.

- Stevia is a good natural sweeter, which is a useful substitute for sugar and it has no known side effects associated with many artificial sweeteners.

- Avoid processed fats like margarines and hydrogenated vegetable oils. You can add healthy fats like coconut oil, olive oil, butter, nut butters and oils.

- Chocolate bars, sweets and candies can be swapped for good quality 80% cocoa chocolate or 100% cocoa powder or cacao nibs can be added to recipes. High cocoa content chocolate may have a small quantity of sugar in it (although less with higher cocoa content) but a small square of chocolate as a treat or recipe addition may be enough of a treat to help you keep eating healthily.

- Where breadcrumbs are needed in recipes, you can grind up some nuts or seeds and use these as a savoury coating instead.

- Cocktails and liqueurs are often loaded with sugar so opt for dry wine instead.

- Swap crisps for vegetable crudités and dip.

- If you check out the ingredients list on processed soups you may realise they should be excluded from your diet due to excess carb/sugar content. Don't let preparation time put you off making your own soups. You can make a large batch and refrigerate or freeze them which will save you time in the long run.

- Be careful of flavoured yogurts – they have large amounts of sugar added. However plain or Greek yogurt is a great addition to your diet and you can get creative by adding, ground nuts, seeds, cocoa powder or a small amount of chopped fruit.

- Pancakes are not off the menu. You can swap ordinary white flour for almond or coconut flour. Or try our really simple recipe for banana pancakes which is so easy you'll wonder why you never thought of it before.

- Although fruit is packed with vitamins and nutrients, it also contains fructose (fruit sugar). So while fruit is beneficial, sugar is not, so keep your intake low and opt for less sugary fruits like raspberries, blueberries and apples. Keep your fruit intake low with no more than 2 pieces per day or less to begin with if you really struggle to balance your blood sugar or have sugar cravings.

Breakfast Recipes

Cloud Bread

Ingredients

50g (2oz) cream cheese

3 eggs

½ teaspoon baking powder

Pinch of salt

MAKES
4

80
calories
each

Method

Line two baking trays with greaseproof paper. Separate the egg yolks from the whites and place them in separate bowls. Add the cream cheese and a pinch of salt to the egg yolks and mix to a smooth batter. In the other bowl, add the baking powder to the egg whites and beat them until they form stiff peaks. Fold the egg yolk mixture into the beaten egg whites and gently combine. Scoop out a large spoonful of the mixture to form a round shape. Transfer them to the oven and bake at 150C/300F for 15-20 minutes until golden. Allow them to cool then store in a plastic bag until ready to use. These delicious bready rolls are a delicious alternative to sandwiches.

Breakfast Bake

Ingredients

SERVES
4

411
calories
per serving

100g (3½ oz) Cheddar cheese, grated (shredded)

50g (2oz) fresh spinach leaves

8 thin sausages

8 eggs, beaten

3 large tomatoes, roughly chopped

1 onion, chopped

2 teaspoon fresh parsley

1 teaspoon paprika

1 tablespoon olive oil

Method

Heat the olive oil in a frying pan, add the sausages and onion into the pan and fry until the sausages are completely cooked. Transfer the sausages and onion to an ovenproof dish. Add in the tomatoes, spinach leaves, eggs, parsley and paprika and mix well. Scatter the grated cheese over the top. Transfer the dish to the oven and bake at 200C/400F for around 35 minutes and the mixture is completely firm.

Savoury Breakfast Muffins

Ingredients

200g (7oz) ham, chopped

75g (3oz) Cheddar cheese, grated (shredded)

8 large eggs, beaten

1 red pepper (bell pepper), finely chopped

1 small courgette (zucchini), finely chopped

MAKES 8

138 calories per serving

Method

Combine the beaten eggs with the ham, cheese, red pepper (bell pepper) and courgette (zucchini). Place paper cases inside a 8–hole muffin tin. Spoon the egg mixture into the cases. Transfer them to the oven and bake at 180C/360F for 20 minutes or until the eggs are completely set. These are so appealing and easy to make in advance to be eaten hot or cold. You can try a variety of fillings and make good use of leftovers, such as chicken, prawns, beef or roast vegetables.

Feta Cheese & Courgette Omelette

Ingredients

25g (1oz) feta cheese, crumbled

2 eggs

1 small courgette (zucchini), grated (shredded)

1 teaspoon fresh parsley, chopped

1 tablespoon olive oil

SERVES
1

337 calories per serving

Method

Place the eggs in a bowl and whisk them. Stir in the cheese and courgette (zucchini). Heat the olive oil in a frying pan. Pour in the egg mixture and cook until it is set. Sprinkle with parsley and serve.

Quinoa & Green Pepper Scramble

Ingredients

100g (3 ½ oz) quinoa, cooked

4 eggs, beaten

1 green pepper (bell pepper), chopped

1 clove of garlic

1 tablespoon olive oil

Sea salt

Freshly ground black pepper

*SERVES
2*

*263
calories
per serving*

Method

Heat the oil in a frying pan, add the garlic and pepper (bell pepper) and cook for 3 minutes. Pour in the beaten eggs and stir continuously until they are almost firm. Add in the quinoa and mix with the egg and green pepper and warm it through. Season with salt and pepper and serve.

Mozzarella & Ham Breakfast Peppers

Ingredients

SERVES 2

160 calories per serving

25g (1oz) mozzarella cheese, grated (shredded)

2 red peppers (bell peppers), cut in half and de-seeded

2 slices ham

2 eggs, beaten

Method

Place a slice of ham into each pepper half. Pour some of the beaten egg into each of the pepper halves. Place the mozzarella on top. Transfer the peppers to a baking sheet and cook in the oven at 190C/375F for 25 minutes or until the eggs have set.

Mediterranean Omelette

Ingredients

50g (2oz) tinned cannellini beans, drained

50g (2oz) mushrooms, chopped

2 eggs

1 red pepper (bell pepper)

1 tablespoon olive oil

Dash of Tabasco sauce or a sprinkle of chilli powder

SERVES 1

394 calories per serving

Method

Heat the olive oil in a pan. Add the mushrooms, pepper (bell pepper) and beans. Cook for 3-4 minutes until the vegetables have softened. Remove them and set aside. Whisk the eggs in a bowl and pour them into the pan. Once the eggs begin to set, return the mushrooms, peppers and beans and spread them onto the eggs. Sprinkle with chilli or Tabasco sauce. Serve and eat straight away.

Avocado Baked Eggs

Ingredients

4 small eggs

2 large avocados, de-stoned and halved

1 tablespoon fresh parsley

¼ teaspoon paprika

SERVES 2

478 calories per serving

Method

Depending on the size you may need to scoop out a little avocado flesh to make room for the egg. Crack the egg into the avocado. Sprinkle with paprika. Place them in an ovenproof dish. Transfer them to the oven and bake at 220C/440F for 18-20 minutes. Sprinkle with parsley and serve.

Creamy Mint Smoothie

Ingredients

SERVES 1

348 calories per serving

250mls (8fl oz) almond milk

8 fresh mint leaves

1 avocado, stone and skin removed

Juice of ½ lime

Method

Place the ingredients into a blender and blitz until smooth. You can add extra almond milk or some water if you like it thinner.

Grapefruit & Kale Smoothie

Ingredients

SERVES 1

230 calories per serving

25g (1oz) kale

1 grapefruit, peeled

2 tablespoons linseeds (flaxseeds)

1 tablespoon sesame seeds

Method

Place all the ingredients into a blender with enough water to cover them and blitz until smooth.

Strawberry & Coconut Smoothie

Ingredients

175ml (6fl oz) full-fat coconut milk

75g (3oz) fresh strawberries

½ avocado, stone and skin removed

SERVES
1

471
calories
per serving

Method

Toss all of the ingredients into a blender. Blitz until creamy and stir in a little water if it seems too thick.

Chicken, Avocado & Basil Omelette

Ingredients

25g (1oz) Cheddar cheese, grated (shredded)

50g (2oz) chicken leftovers, chopped

2 eggs, beaten

Flesh of ½ avocado, chopped

1 teaspoon fresh basil

1 teaspoon olive oil

SERVES 1

491 calories per serving

Method

Heat the olive oil in a frying pan then pour in the beaten egg mixture. While it begins to set sprinkle on the grated cheese, basil, chicken and chopped avocado. Cook until the eggs are completely set and the cheese has melted.

Quinoa Porridge

Ingredients

75g (3oz) quinoa, cooked

50g (2oz) raspberries

1 tablespoon flaked almonds

250mls (8fl oz) unsweetened almond milk

Sprinkling of cinnamon

SERVES 1

262 calories per serving

Method

Pour the almond milk into the saucepan and add in the quinoa and cinnamon. Bring it to the boil and cook for 5 minutes. Serve topped off with the berries and almonds.

Simplest Banana Pancakes

Ingredients

2 eggs

1 banana, mashed

2 teaspoons olive oil

SERVES
1

295
calories
per serving

Method

Whisk the eggs in a bowl and stir in the mashed banana. Combine them until the mixture is smooth. Heat the olive oil in a frying pan, add the pancake mixture and cook for around 2 minutes on each side or until the batter has set and the pancakes are golden. Serve and eat immediately. You can even add a little butter and a sprinkling of cinnamon on top.

Tomato Scrambled Eggs

Ingredients

400g (14oz) tinned chopped tomatoes

4 large eggs, beaten

1 tablespoon olive oil

Sea salt

Freshly ground black pepper

SERVES
2

232
calories
per serving

Method

Heat the olive oil in a pan and add in the chopped tomatoes. Cook for around 10 minutes to reduce the tomato mixture down until the excess juice has evaporated. Slowly pour in the beaten egg, stirring constantly until the egg is completely cooked. Season and serve.

Lunch Recipes

Creamy Tomato Soup

Ingredients

2 x 400g (14oz) tins of chopped tomatoes

25g (1oz) butter

1 red onion, chopped

600mls (1 pint) vegetable stock (broth)

150mls (5fl oz) double cream (heavy cream)

2 tablespoons parsley, minced, optional

Sea salt

Freshly ground black pepper

SERVES
4

293
calories
per serving

Method

Heat the butter in a saucepan, add the onion and cook for 5 minutes. Add in the tomatoes and stock (broth) and bring it to the boil. Reduce the heat and simmer for 5 minutes. Using a food processor and or hand blender blitz until smooth. Pour in the cream and warm it. Sprinkle in the parsley and season with salt and pepper. Serve straight away.

Green Vegetable Soup

Ingredients

SERVES
4

61
calories
per serving

450g (1lb) broccoli, chopped

1 large leek, chopped

1 fennel bulb, chopped

1 courgette (zucchini), chopped

1 handful parsley, chopped

1 handful chives, chopped

Sea salt

Freshly ground black pepper

Method

Place the broccoli, leek, courgette (zucchini) and fennel in enough
water to cover them and bring to the boil. Simmer for 10-15 minutes
or until the vegetables are tender. Stir in the herbs. Using a hand
blender or food processor blend until the soup becomes smooth.
Add more water if required to adjust the consistency. Season and
serve.

Cream of Asparagus Soup

Ingredients

900g (2lbs) asparagus

2 tablespoons crème fraîche

1 onion, chopped

1 tablespoon olive oil

900mls (1½ pints) chicken stock (broth)

Sea salt

Freshly ground black pepper

SERVES 4

104 calories per serving

Method

Heat the oil in a large saucepan, add the onion and cook for 5 minutes. Break off the tough root end of the asparagus and roughly chop it. Place it in the saucepan and add the stock (broth). Bring it to the boil, reduce the heat and simmer for 20 minutes Using a food processor or hand blender process the soup until smooth and creamy. Stir in the crème fraîche. Season and serve.

Cream Of Mushroom Soup

Ingredients

SERVES 4

126 calories per serving

450g (1lb) mushrooms, chopped

1 large leek, finely chopped

1 tablespoon cornflour (cornstarch)

750mls (1¼ pints) vegetable stock (broth)

150mls (5fl oz) crème fraîche

1 tablespoon olive oil

Sea salt

Freshly ground black pepper

Method

Heat the olive oil in a saucepan. Add the leek and mushrooms and cook for 8 minutes or until the vegetables are soft. Sprinkle in the cornflour (cornstarch) and stir. Pour in the stock (broth), bring it to the boil, cover and simmer for 20 minutes. Stir in the crème fraîche. Using a hand blender or food processor, blend the soup until smooth. Return to the heat if necessary. Season with salt and pepper just before serving.

Mozzarella Slices

Ingredients

SERVES 8

157 calories per serving

300g (11oz) mozzarella cheese, grated (shredded)

4 eggs

3 cloves of garlic, crushed

2 teaspoons dried oregano

1 cauliflower (approx 700g), grated (shredded)

Sea salt

Freshly ground black pepper

Method

Steam the cauliflower for 5 minutes or until tender and allow it to cool. Place the cauliflower in a bowl and combine it with the eggs, oregano, garlic and two thirds of the cheese. Season with salt and pepper. Grease 2 baking sheets. Divide the mixture in half and place it on the baking sheet and press it into a flat rectangular shape. Transfer the baking sheets to the oven and bake at 220C/440F for 20-25 minutes or until slightly golden. Remove them from the oven and sprinkle them with the remaining mozzarella cheese. Return them to the oven for 4-5 minutes or until the cheese has melted. Cut into slices and serve.

Szechuan Chicken Salad

Ingredients

450g (1lb) chicken, cut into strips (or turkey)

4 spring onions (scallions), chopped

2 tablespoons fresh coriander (cilantro) leaves, chopped

2 tomatoes, chopped

1 romaine lettuce, chopped

1 cucumber, deseeded and chopped

1 teaspoon ground Szechuan pepper

2 tablespoons sesame oil

Juice of 1 lime

1 tablespoon olive oil

SERVES 4

294 calories per serving

Method

Heat the olive oil in a pan, add the chicken strips and cook for 8 minutes or until the chicken is completely cooked. Remove it and let it cool. Place the chicken, cucumber, tomatoes and coriander (cilantro) in a bowl and stir in the sesame oil, Szechuan pepper, lime juice, spring onions (scallions). Scatter the lettuce on plates and scoop the chicken salad on top.

Fennel & Butterbean Soup

Ingredients

400g (14oz) butter beans

2 large fennel bulbs

1 carrot, chopped

1 onion, chopped

1 courgette (zucchini), chopped

1 clove of garlic, chopped

900mls (1½ pints) vegetable stock (broth)

Sea salt

Freshly ground black pepper

SERVES 4

127 calories per serving

Method

Heat the vegetable stock (broth) in a large saucepan. Add in all of the vegetables but not the butterbeans just yet. Bring them to the boil, reduce the heat and simmer for 20 minutes. Add the butter-beans and stir until warmed through. Using a hand blender or food processor, process the soup until smooth. Season and serve.

Broccoli & Cheddar Soup

Ingredients

SERVES 4

309 calories per serving

175g (6oz) Cheddar cheese, grated (shredded)

1 head of broccoli, chopped

1 leek, chopped

1 courgette (zucchini), chopped

1 litre (1½ pints) chicken stock (broth)

150mls (5fl oz) single cream

Sea salt

Freshly ground black pepper

Method

Place the broccoli, leek and courgette (zucchini) in a saucepan and pour in the stock (broth). Bring them to the boil, reduce the heat and simmer for 15 minutes or until the vegetables are tender. Stir in the cream then using a hand blender or food processor blend until the soup becomes smooth. Add a little hot water or stock (broth) if you want to adjust the consistency. Season with salt and pepper and sprinkle with cheese.

Miso Broth

Ingredients

225g (8oz) pak choi (bok choy), chopped

200g (7oz) tofu, cubed

10 spring onions (scallions), finely chopped

2 star anise

3 tablespoons red miso paste

1 tablespoon fresh coriander (cilantro), freshly chopped

1 cm (½ inch) piece of fresh ginger root, very finely chopped

1 chilli pepper

1200mls (2 pints) vegetable stock (broth)

2 tablespoons soy sauce

SERVES 4

87 calories per serving

Method

Place the pak choi (bok choy) into a saucepan with the ginger, star anise, coriander, chilli and vegetable stock (broth). Bring to the boil, reduce the heat and simmer for 10 minutes. Add the spring onions (scallions), soy sauce and tofu. Cook for 3-4 minutes. In a bowl, mix together the red miso with a few tablespoons of the soup then stir the miso into the soup. Make sure the soup is warmed through. Serve into bowls.

Taco Lettuce Wraps

Ingredients

SERVES
4

386
calories
per serving

450g (1lb) minced beef (ground beef)

100g (3½ oz) cheddar cheese, grated

2 tomatoes, sliced

2 tablespoons tomato purée (paste)

1 romaine or iceberg lettuce, leaves washed and separated

½ teaspoon dried cumin

½ teaspoon paprika

½ teaspoon dried oregano

1 tablespoon olive oil

Method

Heat the olive oil in a frying pan, add the meat, cumin, paprika and oregano and cook for 10 minutes. Add in the tomato purée (paste) and cook for another 5 minutes until the meat is completely cooked. Lay out the lettuce leaves and spoon some meat into each one. Add the tomato slices and sprinkle with cheese. Serve and eat immediately. Your choice of toppings can be varied to include sour cream,

guacamole, mushrooms, onions, chillies or red peppers.

Greek Salad

Ingredients

SERVES 4

176 calories per serving

150g (5oz) cherry tomatoes, halved

75g (3oz) black olives, chopped

50g (2oz) capers

1 romaine lettuce, chopped

1 cucumber chopped

1 red pepper (bell pepper), sliced

1 red onion, sliced

2 tablespoons red wine vinegar

1 tablespoon freshly squeezed lemon juice

½ teaspoon dried oregano

¼ teaspoon dried basil

3 tablespoons olive oil

Sea salt

Freshly ground black pepper

Method

Pour the vinegar into a large bowl and add in the olive oil, lemon juice, basil and oregano and mix well. Season with salt and pepper. Add the tomatoes, olives, capers, lettuce, red pepper (bell pepper) and onion. Toss the salad ingredients in the dressing.

Cheese & Spinach Slice

Ingredients

225g (8oz) mozzarella cheese, grated (shredded)

120g (4oz) ground almonds

25g (1oz) fresh spinach leaves, chopped

2 eggs

1 onion, finely chopped

1 teaspoon baking powder

200mls (7fl oz) almond milk

SERVES
4

390
calories
per serving

Method

Place the spinach into a saucepan, cover it with warm water, bring it to the boil and cook for 3 minutes. Drain it and set aside. Place the ground almonds in a bowl and add in the eggs, milk and baking powder and mix well. Add in the chopped onion, spinach and cheese and combine the mixture. Spoon the mixture into an ovenproof dish and smooth it out. Transfer it to the oven and bake at 190C/375F for 35 minutes. Cut into slices before serving.

Courgette (Zucchini) Fritters

Ingredients

450g (1lb) courgettes (zucchinis), grated (shredded)

100g (3½ oz) Parmesan cheese

3 cloves of garlic

3 spring onions (scallions)

2 eggs

1 teaspoon dried mixed herbs

1 tablespoon olive oil

Sprinkling of salt

SERVES 4

204 calories per serving

Method

Place the grated (shredded) courgette (zucchini) into a colander and sprinkle with a little salt. Allow it to sit for 30 minutes then squeeze out any excess moisture. Place the eggs, Parmesan, spring onions (scallions), garlic and dried herbs into a bowl and mix well with the courgettes. Scoop out a spoonful of the mixture and shape it into patties. Heat the oil in a frying pan, add the patties and cook for 2 minutes, turn them over and cook for another 2 minutes. Serve warm.

Fresh Herb & Feta Salad

Ingredients

**SERVES
2**

**424
calories
per serving**

400g (14oz) tinned cannellini beans, drained

75g (3oz) feta cheese, crumbled or diced

50g (2oz) fresh rocket (arugula) leaves

2 tablespoons fresh basil leaves, chopped

1 tablespoon fresh parsley, chopped

2 tablespoons olive oil

Juice of ½ lemon

Sea salt

Freshly ground black pepper

Method

Place all of the ingredients into a bowl and mix well. Season with salt
and pepper. Chill before serving.

Herby Feta Aubergine (Eggplant) Rolls

Ingredients

SERVES 2

334 calories per serving

125g (4oz) feta cheese

2 tomatoes, chopped

6 asparagus spears

1 aubergine (eggplant) cut into 6 lengthways slices

1 tablespoon fresh basil, chopped

1 tablespoon fresh chives, chopped

2 tablespoons olive oil

Method

Heat the olive oil in a frying pan, add in the aubergine (eggplant) slices and cook for 2-3 minutes on each side. In the meantime, steam the asparagus for 5 minutes until it has softened. Place the aubergine slices onto plates and sprinkle some cheese, tomatoes and herbs onto each slice. Roll the aubergine slices up and secure it with a cocktail stick. Serve and enjoy.

Garlic Dough Balls

Ingredients

125g (4oz) almond flour (ground almonds/ almond meal)

75g (3oz) Parmesan cheese, grated (shredded)

50g (2oz) garlic butter

25g (1oz) mozzarella cheese

25g (1oz) butter, melted

1 egg

1 teaspoon pesto sauce

1 teaspoon garlic powder

MAKES APPROX 20

88 calories per serving

Method

Place all of the ingredients, apart from the garlic butter, into a bowl and combine them. Grease and line a baking tray. Scoop out a tablespoon of the mixture and roll it into a ball. Repeat it for the remaining mixture. Transfer it to the oven and bake at 180C/360F for around 20 minutes, or until golden. Spread some garlic butter onto each dough ball. Enjoy warm.

Prawn & Cannellini Avocados

Ingredients

**SERVES
4**

**333
calories
per serving**

300g (11oz) tinned cannellini beans, drained

300g (11oz) cooked, shelled prawns

2 avocados, halved with stone removed

1 red pepper (bell pepper), finely chopped

2 cloves of garlic, crushed

1 tablespoon fresh coriander (cilantro)

½ teaspoon ground paprika

2 tablespoons extra virgin olive oil

Juice of ½ lemon

Sea salt

Freshly ground black pepper

Method

Pour the lemon juice and olive oil into a bowl and mix well. Stir in the cannellini beans, prawns, red pepper (bell pepper), coriander (cilantro), garlic, paprika, salt and black pepper. Mix together until the ingredients are coated with the dressing. Serve the avocado halves onto plates and scoop the prawn mixture on top.

Bacon & Butterbean Salad

Ingredients

SERVES 2

465 calories per serving

400g (14oz) tin butterbeans, drained

6 strips of bacon, chopped

3 tablespoons red wine vinegar

2 tablespoons fresh chives, chopped

2 tablespoons olive oil

1 teaspoon mustard

Sea salt

Freshly ground black pepper

Method

Heat a frying pan, add the bacon and cook until crispy. Remove it and set it aside to cool. In a bowl, mix together the oil, vinegar, chives and mustard. Stir in the butterbeans and bacon. Season with salt and pepper. Chill before serving.

Parma & Celery Sticks

Ingredients

8 stalks of celery, halved

75g (3oz) cream cheese

4 slices of Parma ham, cut into strips

SERVES
2

248
calories
per serving

Method

Spread some cream cheese onto each celery stick then wrap each one with a slice of ham. Place each one on a baking tray and bake in the oven at 180C/360F for 20 minutes. Serve and eat immediately.

Italian Lentil Salad

Ingredients

SERVES 4

362 calories per serving

450g (1lb) green lentils

100g (3½oz) hazelnuts, chopped

2 spring onions (scallions), chopped

1 cucumber, peeled and diced

1 red pepper (bell pepper), sliced

1 handful of fresh basil

Zest and juice of 1 lemon

100mls (3½ fl oz) extra virgin olive oil

Sea salt

Freshly ground black pepper

Method

Cook the lentils according to the instructions then allow them to cool. Pour the olive oil and lemon juice into a jug and combine them. Season with salt and pepper. Place all the ingredients for the salad into a bowl and pour on the olive oil and lemon juice.

Lemon Lentil Salad

Ingredients

200g (7oz) Puy lentils

4 eggs

4 tomatoes, deseeded and chopped

4 spring onions (scallions), finely chopped

2 tablespoons olive oil

2 tablespoons parsley

2 large handfuls of washed spinach leaves

1 clove of garlic

Juice and rind of 1 lemon

Sea salt

Freshly ground black pepper

SERVES 4

231 calories per serving

Method

Place the lentils in a saucepan, cover them with water and bring them to the boil. Reduce the heat and cook for 20-25 minutes. Drain them once they are soft. Heat the olive oil in a saucepan, add the garlic and spring onions (scallions) and cook for 2 minutes. Stir in the tomatoes, lemon juice and rind. Cook for 2 minutes. Stir in the lentils and keep warm. In a pan of gently simmering water, poach the eggs until they are set but soft in the middle which should be 3-4 minutes. Scatter the spinach leaves onto plates, serve the lentils and top off with a poached egg. Season with salt and pepper.

Halloumi & Asparagus Salad

Ingredients

450g (1lb) asparagus

250g (9oz) halloumi cheese, cut into slices

2 large handfuls of spinach leaves

1 tablespoon olive oil

Sea salt

Freshly ground black pepper

SERVES 4

257 calories per serving

Method

Heat the olive oil in a frying pan and cook the asparagus for 4 minutes or until tender. Remove, set aside and keep warm. Place the halloumi in the frying pan and cook for 2 minutes on each side until golden. Serve the spinach leaves onto plates and add the asparagus and halloumi slices. Season with salt and pepper.

Chicken & Quinoa Salad

Ingredients

SERVES 4

296 calories per serving

450g (1lb) chicken breasts, cooked and sliced

125g (4oz) quinoa, cooked

50g (2oz) fresh spinach leaves, chopped

8 spring onions (scallions), chopped

1 handful fresh coriander (cilantro), chopped

1 handful fresh parsley, chopped

2 tomatoes, diced

1 cucumber, peeled and diced

1 teaspoon ground turmeric

2 tablespoons olive oil

Juice of 1 lime

Sea salt

Freshly ground black pepper

Method

Combine all of the ingredients in a large bowl and mix well. Season with salt and pepper. Cover and place in the fridge for 20 minutes to chill before serving.

Goat's Cheese & Olive Salad

Ingredients

SERVES 4

264 calories per serving

350g (12oz) tomatoes, de-seeded and chopped

150g (5oz) goat's cheese, crumbled

50g (2oz) pitted black olives, chopped

1 romaine lettuce, finely chopped

1 cucumber, de-seeded and chopped

DRESSING:

3 tablespoons olive oil

Juice of 1 lemon

Sea salt

Freshly ground black pepper

Method

In a bowl, mix together the dressing ingredients. Place all of the salad ingredients into a bowl and add in the dressing. Toss the salad well before serving.

Aubergine (Eggplant) Fries

Ingredients

SERVES 4

255 calories per serving

125g (4oz) ground almonds (almond meal/almond flour)

1 large egg

1 large aubergine (eggplant), cut lengthwise into batons

½ teaspoon salt

½ teaspoon ground cumin

½ teaspoon paprika

1 tablespoon olive oil

Sea salt

Freshly ground black pepper

Method

Place the ground almonds on a large plate and season with salt and pepper. In a bowl, beat the egg and stir in the cumin and paprika. Dip the aubergine batons in egg then roll them in the almond mixture. Place the aubergine on a baking sheet. Transfer it to the oven and cook at 220C/425F for 15 minutes.

Chilli Cheese Crisps

Ingredients

100g (3 ½ oz) Cheddar cheese, grated (shredded)

1 green chilli pepper, de-seeded and thinly sliced

SERVES 4

104 calories per serving

Method

Line a baking sheet with greaseproof paper. Scoop a tablespoon of the grated (shredded) cheese and place the mound of cheese onto the paper then press it down slightly, keeping a circular shape. Place a thin slice of chilli on top. Repeat for the remaining mixture. Transfer to the oven and cook at 180C/360F for 12 minutes until the cheese has melted. Remove them from the oven and allow them to cool before removing them from the paper.

Baked Aubergine (Eggplant) & Garlic Dip

Ingredients

125g (4oz) plain yogurt

50g (2oz) cucumber, grated (shredded)

2 aubergines (eggplants) cut into slices

1 clove of garlic, crushed

1 tablespoon olive oil

Sea salt

Freshly ground black pepper

SERVES 4

83 calories per serving

Method

Pour the olive oil onto a baking tray and place the aubergine (eggplants) on the tray. Transfer the tray to the oven and book at 180C/360F for 40 minutes. In the meantime prepare the dip. Combine the yogurt, cucumber and garlic. Season with salt and pepper. Serve the aubergine (eggplant) with a dollop of yogurt.

Dinner Recipes

Pork Steaks, Peppers & Beans

Ingredients

400g (14oz) cannellini beans, drained

8 pork steaks

4 tablespoons fresh parsley, chopped

2 red peppers (bell peppers)

1 onion, chopped

1 tablespoon red wine vinegar

1 tablespoon olive oil

Sea salt

Freshly ground black pepper

**SERVES
4**

**460
calories
per serving**

Method

Season the pork steaks with salt and pepper. Heat the olive oil in a frying pan, add the pork and cook for around 3 minutes on each side. Remove them, set aside and keep them warm. Add the peppers (bell peppers) and onion to the pan and cook for 5 minutes until the vegetables have softened. Add the parsley, vinegar and beans and warm them thoroughly. Serve the pork steaks and spoon the vegetables over the top. Enjoy.

Fresh Basil, Mozzarella & Tomato Chicken

Ingredients

4 chicken breasts

2 x 400g (14oz) tins of chopped tomatoes

125g (4oz) mozzarella cheese, sliced

600mls (1 pint) vegetable stock (broth)

1 large handful of fresh basil leaves, torn

2 cloves of garlic

1 onion chopped

1 tablespoon olive oil

SERVES 4

324 calories per serving

Method

Heat the olive oil in a frying pan, add the onion and garlic and cook for 5 minutes or until softened. Add the chopped tomatoes and stock (broth). Add in the basil leaves, bring it to the boil, reduce the heat and simmer for 5 minutes. Place the chicken in an ovenproof dish. Cover the chicken with the sauce and add slices of mozzarella to the dish. Transfer it to the oven and cook at 190C/375F for around 20 minutes or until the chicken is completely cooked. Serve with a leafy green salad.

Baked Eggs & Vegetables

Ingredients

4 eggs

1 red pepper (bell pepper), chopped

1 green pepper (bell pepper), chopped

1 large aubergine (eggplant), chopped

1 bulb of fennel, chopped

1 onion, chopped

3 cloves of garlic, chopped

1 handful of fresh basil

2 tablespoons olive oil

*SERVES
4*

*174
calories
per serving*

Method

Place all the vegetables, garlic and basil in a large ovenproof dish. Pour in the olive oil and toss the vegetables. Transfer it to the oven and cook at 200C/400F for 20 minutes. Make 4 round indentations in the vegetables and crack an egg into each space. Place the dish back into the oven and cook for 10 minutes. Serve and eat immediately.

Beef Stir-Fry

Ingredients

450g (1lb) beef steak, cut into strips

350g (12oz) broccoli, broken into florets then halve them

175g (6oz) mushrooms, sliced

3 cloves of garlic, crushed

1 pak choi (bok choy), chopped

1 red pepper (bell pepper)

2 tablespoons olive oil

2.5cm (1 inch) chunk of fresh root ginger, chopped

2 tablespoons soy sauce

1 teaspoon Chinese five-spice

Sea salt

Freshly ground black pepper

SERVES
4

326
calories
per serving

Method

Heat a tablespoon of olive oil in a large frying pan or wok until it begins to smoke. Add the beef and brown it then remove and set aside. Heat the remaining olive oil and mushrooms, ginger, five-spice and garlic and cook for 3 minutes. Add in the broccoli and red pepper (bell pepper) and cook for 4 minutes. Stir in the pak choi (bok choy) and cook until softened. Add the beef strips and stir in the soy sauce. Season with salt and pepper. Serve and enjoy.

Cauliflower Mash

Ingredients

1 large head of cauliflower, approx.700g (1½ lb), broken into florets

75g (3oz) Cheddar cheese, grated (shredded)

75g (3oz) crème fraîche

1 clove of garlic, crushed

SERVES
6

107 calories per serving

Method

Place the cauliflower in a steamer along with the garlic and cook until the cauliflower has softened. Drain it and allow it to cool just a little. Transfer it to a food processor and process until smooth. Stir in the crème fraîche and cheese and mix it well. Serve instead of traditional mashed potatoes.

Mustard & Garlic Prawns

Ingredients

450g (1lb) large fresh uncooked prawns, peeled

125g (4oz) butter

2 red peppers (bell peppers), sliced

2 tablespoons Dijon mustard

Juice of half a lemon

2 cloves of garlic, chopped

Sea salt

Freshly ground black pepper

SERVES 4

331 calories per serving

Method

Place the prawns in an ovenproof dish and scatter the red peppers (bell peppers) into the dish. Heat the butter in a small saucepan and stir in the mustard, garlic and lemon juice. Warm the mixture until the butter has melted. Pour the butter over the prawns and peppers. Season with salt and pepper. Transfer to the oven and bake at 220C/425F for 15 minutes or until the prawns are pink and completely cooked.

Marinated Pork Chops

Ingredients

4 pork chops

100mls (3½ fl oz) soy sauce

4 cloves garlic, minced

2 teaspoons ground coriander (cilantro)

½ teaspoon ground black pepper

2 tablespoons extra virgin olive oil

Juice of ½ lemon

SERVES 4

320 calories per serving

Method

Place the garlic, soy sauce, lemon juice, olive oil, coriander (cilantro) and pepper in a bowl and mix well. Add the pork chops to the bowl and coat them thoroughly in the mixture. Cover and refrigerate them for at least 30 minutes, or overnight if you can. When they are sufficiently marinated, heat a frying pan and add the chops together with all of the marinade. Cook for 5 minutes on each side, or until the chops are thoroughly cooked. Serve with a heap of green salad and courgette 'spaghetti'.

Slow Cooked Chicken

Ingredients

1 large whole chicken, approx. 1.8kg (4 lb)

1 red onion, halved

1 teaspoon paprika (you can use smoked paprika as an alternative)

Sea salt

Freshly ground black pepper

SERVES 6

423 calories per serving

Method

Sprinkle the paprika over the chicken and season with salt and pepper. Place the onion inside the chicken. Transfer it to a slow cooker and cook on high for 6-8 hours or until the chicken is completely cooked and very tender. Serve the chicken with the juices spooned over the top and a heap of fresh vegetables.

Cottage Pie

Ingredients

450g (1lb) beef mince (ground beef)

400g (14oz) tinned chopped tomatoes

1 carrot, peeled and finely chopped

1 cauliflower (approx.700g (1½ lb) broken into florets

1 leek, trimmed and finely chopped

1 onion, chopped

1 tablespoon soy sauce

1 tablespoon tomato purée (paste)

1 tablespoon olive oil

1 small handful fresh parsley, chopped

300mls (½ pint) beef stock (broth)

SERVES
4

370
calories
per serving

Method

Heat the oil in a saucepan, add the mince and cook for 3 minutes. Add in the carrot and onion and cook for 5 minutes. Add in the tomatoes, tomato purée, soy sauce, parsley and stock (broth). Bring it to the boil, reduce the heat and simmer for 30 minutes. In the meantime, boil the cauliflower until tender then drain it. Mash until soft. Fry the leeks in a pan until they become soft. Combine the leeks with the mashed cauliflower. Transfer the meat to an ovenproof dish and spoon the cauliflower mixture on top. Place the dish in the oven at 200C/400F for around 30 minutes or golden on top.

Lamb Shank Casserole

Ingredients

SERVES
2

432
calories
per serving

2 lamb shanks

4 large mushrooms, chopped

3 carrots, chopped

3 cloves of garlic, crushed

2 large tomatoes, chopped

1 onion, finely chopped

2 tablespoons tomato purée (paste)

2 large sprigs of rosemary

1 bouquet garni

½ bulb of fennel, chopped

750mls (1¼ pints) beef vegetable stock (broth)

2 tablespoons olive oil

Method

Heat the oil in a large saucepan and add the lamb, turning occasionally until it is brown all over. Transfer the lamb to a bowl and set aside. Add the onion, fennel, mushrooms, carrots and garlic to the saucepan and cook for 5 minutes. Return the lamb to the saucepan and add in the stock, tomatoes, tomato purée (paste), rosemary, and bouquet garni. Transfer to an oven-proof dish, cover and cook in the oven at 200C/400F for 2 hours. Check half way through cooking and add extra stock (broth) or water if necessary. Remove the bouquet garni. Serve and enjoy.

Harissa Meatballs & Yogurt Dip

Ingredients

450g (1lb) minced turkey (or beef)

50g (2oz) ground almonds

3 tablespoons harissa paste

1 tablespoon tomato purée (paste)

1 garlic clove, crushed

Juice of 1 lemon

1 egg

2 tablespoons extra virgin olive oil

FOR THE DIP:

200g (7oz) plain yogurt (unflavoured)

12 mint leaves, finely chopped

SERVES
4

*344
calories
per serving*

Method

In a bowl, combine the turkey with 2 tablespoons of harissa paste, the almonds, garlic, lemon juice and egg and mix really well. Scoop portions of the mixture out with a spoon and shape into balls. Cover and refrigerate for 40 minutes. Heat the oil in a frying pan, add a tablespoon of harissa paste and tomato purée (paste) and stir. Add the meatballs and cook for 7-8 minutes, turning occasionally until thoroughly cooked. In the meantime, combine the yogurt and mint and mix well. Skewer each meatball with a cocktail stick and serve ready to be dipped in the yogurt. Enjoy.

Low-Carb Turkey Lasagne

Ingredients

SERVES 6

443 calories per serving

450g (1lb) minced (ground) turkey
400g (14oz) ricotta cheese
300g (11oz) mozzarella cheese, grated (shredded)
2 x 400g (14oz) tin of chopped tomatoes
25g (1oz) Parmesan cheese
4 courgettes (zucchinis) sliced lengthways
3 tablespoons fresh basil, chopped
2 cloves of garlic, crushed
1 onion, chopped
1 red pepper (bell pepper), chopped
1 teaspoon dried oregano
1 egg
1 tablespoon olive oil

Method

Grease a baking sheet and lay the courgette (zucchini) slices on it. Season with salt, transfer it to the oven and bake at 190C/375F for 15 minutes. In the meantime, heat the oil in a saucepan, add the onions, garlic and red pepper (bell pepper) and cook for 5 minutes. Add in the turkey and cook for 4 minutes. Stir in the tomatoes, basil and oregano. Bring it to the boil, reduce the heat and simmer for 30 minutes. In a bowl combine the egg and ricotta cheese then set aside. When the turkey mixture is cooked, spoon half of it into an ovenproof dish. Add a layer of the baked courgettes then spoon on half of the ricotta mixture and a layer of mozzarella, repeat with the remaining mixture. Sprinkle Parmesan on top. Transfer it to the oven and bake at 375F/180C for 40 minutes. Serve with a leafy green salad.

Lemon & Herb Lamb Chops

Ingredients

12 small lamb chops

1 tablespoon fresh thyme, chopped

½ tablespoon fresh rosemary leaves

4 tablespoons extra virgin olive oil

Juice of 1 lemon

*SERVES
4*

*307
calories
per serving*

Method

Pour the oil into a bowl and stir in the lemon juice, rosemary and thyme. Place the lamb chops in the mixture and allow it to marinate for at least 1 hour or overnight if you can. Transfer the chops to a hot grill (broiler) and cook for 5 minutes on either side or until the chops are cooked to your liking. Serve with courgette 'spaghetti' and a salad.

Salmon, Butter Beans & Yogurt Dressing

Ingredients

400g (14oz) butter beans

125g (4oz) plain Greek yogurt (full-fat)

4 salmon fillets

3 cloves of garlic

1 red chilli, finely chopped

½ teaspoon paprika, plus extra for seasoning

½ teaspoon oregano

1 tablespoon olive oil

Zest and juice ½ lemon

Sea salt

Freshly ground black pepper

SERVES 4

385 calories per serving

Method

Place the yogurt into a bowl and add in the lemon juice and paprika. Heat the oil in a pan, add the oregano, garlic and chilli and warm them for 2 minutes. Add in the butter beans and lemon zest and warm them through. Sprinkle the paprika over the salmon and season it with salt and pepper. Place the salmon fillets under a hot grill (broiler) and cook for around 8 minutes, or until completely cooked, turning half way through. Serve the salmon with the butter beans and a dollop of yogurt dressing.

Hunters Chicken

Ingredients

SERVES 4

476 calories per serving

400g (14oz) broccoli florets

125g (4oz) cheese, grated (shredded)

8 slices of bacon

4 chicken breasts

1 onion, chopped

250g (8oz) tomato passata (sauce)

3 tablespoons balsamic vinegar

1 tablespoon olive oil

Method

Heat the oil in a frying pan, add the onion and cook for 5 minutes. Add the passata and balsamic and cook for 10 minutes to reduce the mixture. Place the chicken flat-side down on a lightly greased ovenproof and make an incision to make room for the sauce. Spoon the sauce into the incision. Wrap two slices of bacon around each chicken breast. Transfer the chicken to the oven and cook for 25 minutes. Scatter the cheese over the chicken breasts and return them to the oven for 5 minutes or until the cheese is bubbling. In the meantime steam or boil the broccoli for 5 minutes. Serve the broccoli onto plates and add the chicken.

Mediterranean Fish Casserole

Ingredients

4 tuna steaks

2 red onions, chopped

2 stalks of celery

2 x 400g (2 x 14oz) tins of chopped tomatoes

2 cloves of garlic

1 tablespoon olive oil

1 lemon, thinly sliced

1 tablespoon tomato purée (paste)

2 tablespoons fresh oregano, chopped

Sea salt

Freshly ground black pepper

SERVES 4

229 calories per serving

Method

Heat the oil in a saucepan and add the celery, garlic and onions and fry for 5 until the vegetables have softened. Add in the tinned tomatoes, oregano, tomato puree (paste) and lemon slices. Bring to the boil and simmer, stirring, for 5 minutes. Season with salt and pepper. Place the fish in the tomato mixture. Simmer gently for 12-14 min-

utes until the fish is cooked. Serve the fish onto plates and pour the

Tomato & Herb Stuffed Chicken

Ingredients

450g (1lb) chicken breasts

75g (3oz) black olives, finely chopped

50g (2oz) butter, softened

6 sundried tomatoes, finely chopped

3 cloves of garlic, crushed

1 tablespoon capers

1 teaspoon dried oregano

1 teaspoon dried basil

Sea salt

Freshly ground black pepper

SERVES 4

333 calories per serving

Method

Place the olives, tomatoes, garlic, dried herbs and capers into a bowl and stir. Add in the softened butter and capers and mix well. Make an incision in each chicken breast to make a pocket for the butter mixture. Spoon the mixture inside each of the chicken breasts. Season with salt and pepper and wrap each one in tin foil. Transfer them to the oven and cook at 190C/375F for 25 minutes.

Lemon & Coriander (Cilantro) Chicken

Ingredients

450g (1lb) chicken breasts

1 onion, finely chopped

3 cloves of garlic, crushed

2 lemons, sliced and pips removed

1 teaspoon ground coriander

1 teaspoon ground ginger

1 teaspoon ground cumin

1 teaspoon ground turmeric

1 tablespoon extra virgin olive oil

600mls (1 pint) chicken stock (broth)

125g (4oz) pitted green olives

Handful of fresh coriander (cilantro) finely chopped

SERVES 4

278 calories per serving

Method

Heat the oil in a saucepan, add the onion and cook for 5 minutes until softened. Add the garlic, cumin, turmeric, ginger and ground coriander (cilantro) and cook for 1 minute. Add the chicken and brown it. Add the slices of lemon and chicken stock (broth). Bring it to the boil, reduce the heat and simmer for 30 minutes. Stir in the fresh coriander (cilantro) and olives. Warm the olives through and then serve.

Golden Cauliflower 'Rice'

Ingredients

1 head of cauliflower, approx 700g (1½ lb)

1 tablespoon olive oil

Sea salt

Freshly ground black pepper

SERVES 4

81 calories per serving

Method

Place the cauliflower into a food processor and chop until fine, similar to rice. Heat the olive oil in a frying pan, stir in the cauliflower and cook for 5-6 minutes or until softened. Season with salt and pepper. Serve with meat or vegetable dishes as a tasty alternative to rice.

Vegetable Fried 'Rice'

Ingredients

SERVES 4

199 calories per serving

200g (7oz) beansprouts

6 spring onions (scallions), finely chopped

1 head of cauliflower, approx 700g (1½ lb) broken into florets

1 carrot, peeled and finely chopped

1 red onion, finely chopped

1 large egg, beaten

2 tablespoons olive oil

2 tablespoons soy sauce

Sea salt

Freshly ground black pepper

Method

Place the cauliflower pieces into a food processor and chop until it becomes grain-like. In a bowl mix together the egg with a tablespoon of soy sauce. Heat a tablespoon of oil in a large frying pan or wok. Add the egg mixture and scramble it for a few minutes then remove it and set aside. Heat the remaining olive oil and add in the red onion and cook for 5 minutes. Add in all the remaining vegetables and cook them for around 5 minutes until they soften. Stir in the remaining soy sauce. Add the cooked egg mixture and stir well. Season with salt and pepper. Serve instead of traditional fried rice.

Quinoa & Coriander (Cilantro) Cakes

Ingredients

100g (3½oz) quinoa, cooked

50g (2oz) Cheddar cheese, grated (shredded)

25g (1oz) ground almonds

4 tablespoons fresh coriander (cilantro), chopped

2 eggs, beaten

1 onion, finely chopped

½ teaspoon turmeric

1 tablespoon olive oil

Sea salt

Freshly ground black pepper

SERVES 2

328 calories per serving

Method

In a bowl, combine the eggs, onion, coriander (cilantro), turmeric, cheese, almonds and season with salt and pepper. Stir in the quinoa and mix well. With clean hands, form 8 small patties. Heat the olive oil in a frying pan and add the quinoa cakes. Cook for 3-4 minutes on either side until slightly golden.

Salmon Kebabs

Ingredients

8 button mushrooms

8 pitted black olives

4 salmon fillets

2 tablespoons fresh parsley, chopped

Juice and rind of 1 lemon

3 tablespoons olive oil

**SERVES
4**

*385
calories
per serving*

Method

Cut the salmon into chunks and place them in a bowl. Squeeze in the lemon juice and add the rind, olive oil and parsley and coat the salmon chunks thoroughly. Add the mushrooms and coat them in the dressing too. Thread the fish, olives and mushrooms onto skewers. Place them under a hot grill (broiler) and cook for 4-5 minutes turning occasionally. Serve the kebabs and drizzle them with the remaining dressing.

Coconut & Vegetable Curry

Ingredients

200g (7oz) tofu, cubed

200g (7oz) mushrooms, chopped

125g (4oz) green beans, chopped

2 tablespoons fresh coriander (cilantro), chopped

1 tablespoon medium curry powder

1 teaspoon cumin

1 teaspoon turmeric

1 teaspoon ground ginger

400mls (14fl oz) full-fat coconut milk

Sea salt

Freshly ground black pepper

SERVES 4

207 calories per serving

Method

Warm the coconut milk in a saucepan then add in the curry powder, cumin, ginger and turmeric and mix it well. Add the mushrooms, green beans, tofu and stir. Bring it to the boil, reduce the heat and simmer for 8-10 minutes until the vegetables are soft. Sprinkle with coriander (cilantro) and serve with cauliflower rice.

Spinach & Cheese Stuffed Chicken

Ingredients

4 chicken breasts

4 tablespoons cream cheese

25g (1oz) spinach leaves

1 tablespoon fresh parsley

1 tablespoon fresh chives

SERVES 4

192 calories per serving

Method

In a bowl, combine the cream cheese, spinach and herbs until it's well mixed. Carefully make an incision on the underside of the chicken breast, wide enough to contain some cheese mixture. Spoon some of the mixture into the incision and press the chicken back together. Repeat for the remaining mixture. Place the stuffed chicken in an ovenproof dish. Transfer to the oven and bake at 180C/360F for around 30 minutes or until the chicken is completely cooked. Serve with a large green leafy salad. Enjoy.

Marinated Spare Ribs

Ingredients

1kg (2lb 4oz) pork ribs, individually cut

3 teaspoons paprika

1 teaspoon ground ginger

½ teaspoon cinnamon

½ teaspoon ground star anise

¼ teaspoon salt

½ teaspoon white pepper

3 tablespoons olive oil

*SERVES
4*

*334
calories
per serving*

Method

Place the spices, salt, pepper and oil in a bowl and combine. Coat the ribs with the spice mixture and coat them thoroughly. Cover them and allow them to marinate for 30 minutes or overnight if you can. Place the pork ribs in a roasting tin, transfer them to the oven and cook at 180C/360F for 35-40 minutes. Serve onto a large plate for sharing.

Coriander & Coconut Baked Salmon

Ingredients

4 salmon fillets,

120mls (4fl oz) coconut milk

1 large handful of coriander (cilantro) leaves

2.5cm (1 inch) chunk of ginger

1 teaspoon garam masala

3 cloves of garlic, crushed

1 chilli pepper, de-seeded and chopped

SERVES 4

228 calories per serving

Method

Pour the coconut milk into a blender and add in the ginger, garam masala, garlic, chilli and coriander (cilantro). Process until smooth. Place the salmon fillets in an ovenproof dish and pour the coconut milk over the fish. Transfer it to the oven and bake at 220C/440F for 15-20 minutes until the fish is cooked through.

Roast Courgettes (Zucchinis) & Olives

Ingredients

10 pitted black olives, chopped

4 medium courgettes (zucchinis), thickly sliced lengthways

2 tablespoons tomato purée (paste)

1 clove of garlic, crushed

1 teaspoon mixed herbs

2 tablespoons olive oil

Sea salt

Freshly ground black pepper

SERVES 4

107 calories per serving

Method

In a bowl, combine the olive oil, garlic, tomato purée (paste) and mixed herbs. Place the courgette (zucchini) slices in an ovenproof dish and spread the oil mixture over the slices. Sprinkle with olives and season with salt and pepper. Transfer them to an oven, preheated to 200C/400F and cook for 15 minutes.

Mini Cauliflower Pizza Bases

Ingredients

SERVES 6

219 calories per serving

350g (12 oz) mozzarella cheese, grated (shredded)

2 eggs

1 head of cauliflower approx 700g (1½ lb), grated (shredded)

1 teaspoon dried oregano

1 teaspoon dried basil

1 teaspoon garlic powder

1 tomato, sliced

Handful of fresh basil leaves, chopped

200g (7oz) passata/ tomato sauce

Method

Steam the grated (shredded) cauliflower for 5 minutes then allow it to cool. Place the cooked cauliflower in a bowl and add the eggs, half the cheese, all of the dried herbs and garlic and mix everything together really well. Grease two baking sheets. Divide the mixture into 12 and roll it into balls. Place them on a baking sheet and press them down until flat and round mini pizza bases. Transfer them to the oven and bake at 220C/440F for 12 minutes until lightly golden. Top each pizza base with a little passata, the remaining mozzarella and tomato and basil. Place the pizzas under a grill (broiler) and cook for 4-5 minutes or until the cheese has melted. Enjoy.

Parmesan Chicken

Ingredients

SERVES 4

279 calories per serving

4 large chicken breasts, cut into strips

75g (3oz) Parmesan cheese, grated (shredded)

1 teaspoon dried oregano

1 teaspoon paprika

1 teaspoon white pepper

1 large egg, beaten

1 tablespoon extra virgin olive oil

Method

On a plate, combine the Parmesan cheese with the oregano, paprika and pepper. Dip the chicken strips in the beaten egg and then coat them liberally with the Parmesan mixture. Heat the olive oil in a frying pan, add the chicken strips and cook them for around 4 or 5 minutes on each side, or until they are completely cooked.

Mediterranean Cod

Ingredients

4 cod fillets

1 onion, chopped

2 cloves of garlic, crushed

1 x 400g (14oz) tin of chopped tomatoes

75g (3oz) pitted black olives, sliced

2 tablespoons olive oil

100mls (3½ fl oz) vegetable or chicken stock (broth)

Handful of fresh parsley

SERVES 4

223 calories per serving

Method

Heat the oil in a frying pan, add the onions and garlic and cook for 5 minutes. Add in chopped tomatoes, parsley, olives and stock. Bring it to the boil and simmer for 5 minutes. Add the cod fillets in the sauce and simmer gently for 5-6 minutes or until the fish is white and thoroughly cooked.

Desserts & Snacks

Pistachio Brownies

Ingredients

125g (4oz) cream cheese

50g (2oz) coconut oil, melted

50g (2oz) butter, melted

75g (3oz) shelled pistachio nuts, chopped

3 tablespoons 100% cocoa powder

6 eggs

2 teaspoons vanilla extract

2 tablespoons stevia sweetener (or to taste)

½ teaspoon baking powder

MAKES 16

155 calories per serving

Method

Place all of the ingredients (except the nuts) into a bowl and combine the mixture thoroughly. Stir in the pistachio nuts. Scoop the mixture into a lined baking tray and spread it out evenly. Transfer it to the oven and bake at 180C/360F for around 20 minutes or until cooked through. Allow it to cool before slicing into portions.

Raspberry Muffins

Ingredients

MAKES 10

222 calories per serving

250g (9oz) ground almonds (almond flour/almond meal)

150g (5oz) fresh raspberries

3 eggs, whisked

1 teaspoon baking powder

1 teaspoon stevia powder (or to taste)

50mls (2fl oz) melted coconut oil

Pinch of salt

Method

Lightly grease a 10-hole muffin tin. In a bowl, combine the ground almonds (almond flour/almond meal), baking powder, stevia and salt. In another bowl, combine the coconut oil and eggs then pour the mixture into the dry ingredients. Mix well. Add the raspberries to the mixture and gently stir them in. Spoon some of the mixture into each of the muffin moulds. Transfer them to the oven and bake at 170C/325F for around 20 minutes or until golden.

Chocolate Muesli Bites

Ingredients

MAKES 24

128 calories per serving

125g (4oz) walnuts, chopped

125g (4oz) almonds, chopped

50g (2oz) desiccated (shredded) coconut

50g (2oz) coconut oil

2 eggs, beaten

2 tablespoons 100% cocoa powder (or cacao nibs)

2 tablespoons tahini paste

2 tablespoons peanut butter

1 tablespoon sunflower seeds

1 teaspoon ground cinnamon

1 tablespoon stevia

Method

Place all the ingredients into a bowl or a food processor and mix it well, keeping the nuts a nice chunky texture. Spoon the mixture into paper baking cases. Transfer them to the oven and bake at 180C/360F for 20 minutes. Allow them to cool then store them in an airtight container.

Baked Chocolate Cheesecake

Ingredients

800g (1¾ lb) mascarpone cheese

4 medium eggs, beaten

3 tablespoons 100% cocoa powder

1-2 tablespoon stevia sweetener (or to taste)

SERVES 10

391 calories per serving

Method

Place the mascarpone cheese into a bowl and beat it until soft. Stir in the eggs, cocoa powder and stevia and mix well. Transfer the mixture to an ovenproof dish and bake in the oven at 170C/325F for one hour. Remove it and allow it to cool before serving.

Quick Lemon Cake

Ingredients

2 tablespoons ground almonds (almond flour/almond meal)

2 tablespoons ground flax seeds (linseeds)

2 eggs

1 tablespoon butter

1 teaspoon stevia powder (or to taste)

½ teaspoon baking powder

1 tablespoon lemon juice

½ teaspoon lemon zest

SERVES 2

287 calories per serving

Method

Place the butter in a large mug or glass dish and warm it in the microwave until melted. Crack the eggs into the mug/dish and whisk them together with the lemon zest and juice. Stir in the almonds, ground flax seeds (linseeds), baking powder and stevia and mix well. Microwave the mug/dish on high for around 2 minutes or until the mixture has risen.

High Protein Chocolate Balls

Ingredients

MAKES 12

102 calories per ball

75g (3oz) peanut butter

25g (1oz) coconut oil

50g (2oz) desiccated (shredded) coconut

25g (1oz) chia seeds

2 teaspoons coconut flour

1 tablespoon 100% cocoa powder

1 tablespoon stevia sweetener

Cocoa powder for coating (approx 1 tablespoon)

Method

Place all the ingredients into a bowl or food processor (apart from the cocoa powder for coating) and process until smooth. Using a teaspoon, scoop out a little of the mixture, shape it into a ball and roll it in cocoa powder. Chill before serving.

Strawberry Ice-Cream

Ingredients

600mls (1 pint) coconut milk

300g (11oz) ripe strawberries

2 ripe bananas

SERVES 4

296 calories per serving

Method

Place all the ingredients into a food processor and until smooth and creamy. Transfer the mixture to an ice-cream maker and process according to the instructions for your machine. If you don't have an ice cream maker, place it in the freezer and occasionally whisk it with a fork every couple of hours whilst it is freezing.

Hot Chocolate

Ingredients

300mls (½ pint) almond milk

¼ teaspoon cinnamon

1 teaspoon 100% cocoa powder

Stevia sweetener to taste

SERVES 1

93 calories per serving

Method

Place the almond milk, cinnamon and cocoa powder in a saucepan and whisk them together. Bring it to almost boiling, remove it from the heat and whisk a little more. Check the sweetness and add a little extra sweetener and/or cinnamon. Enjoy.

Printed in Great Britain
by Amazon